Essential Tips
for
Beginning Martial Artists

By Pat Smith

I0419865

Introduction

So you want to become a martial artist, or perhaps you already are one. Then this booklet is for you. Even if you've spent the better part of a decade studying the martial arts, you'll probably be able to benefit from the tips I have included here for beginners.

These tips have come from my extensive nearly thirty years' of martial arts experience. Most martial arts experts excel in one area or another. On rare occasions they excel in more than one. Some are true masters of the style in which they've spent countless hours each day training for decades. Others are masterful teachers. Others succeed in Hollywood, or by some other means, and become famous popularizing the martial arts in general. Others excel in competition, in the Olympics or in the Ultimate Fighting Championship.

I don't claim to be any of the above. Then why read my booklet? Because the secrets I'm going to share here I either learned from masters in each of the above categories, or else I learned the hard way through making many mistakes. I want everyone interested in the martial arts to avoid the mistakes I made, and also learn the wisdom I gained from my elite instructors which have included world champion full contact fighters, Grandmasters and founders of their own styles, top trainers of world champions, as well as an elite hand-to-hand combat instructor of special forces from the U.S. and from abroad (e.g., Australia, England, Germany, and Israel).

The chances of you ever working with any instructor of this caliber, outside of occasional seminars, is highly unlikely, because they tend not to take on large numbers of students. Exceptions exist, especially when it comes to fighting champions.

In this booklet, however, I want to impart some of these golden nuggets of wisdom that have taken me nearly three decades to learn. I promise that if you put these lessons into practice, you will avoid most of the mistakes I have made, and you will accelerate your martial arts practice and skills, REGARDLESS of your goal or the style you train.

Let's face it, people come to the martial arts for an incredible diverse array of reasons. Some want to learn how to defend themselves, against bullies at school, against potential dangers in our very dangerous society, or because they have already been traumatized and want to ensure to the best of their abilities, that that will never happen again.

Others simply want to get in better shape and recognize that the martial arts, regardless of style, is a great way to get in better physical shape. Others want to learn to be more self-disciplined. Others want to win martial arts competitions, become the next Ultimate Fighting Champion. Some others seek a profession in the stunt business, or else are training for particular acting requirements. Others want to gain self-confidence.

Often there is a combination of reasons for beginning martial arts training. Some individuals, and this is my story, begin from a specific motive, like self-defense, and then fall in love with the martial arts and want to dedicate their lives to studying the art, as an art, and as a way of life. For any of these reasons, this booklet is for you.

Occasionally, someone will come to the martial arts because they want to hurt people, to bully, to acquire a dangerous power or skill in order to use it maliciously against others. If that is your motive, then I recommend you stay away from the martial arts, and I'll let you know up front that this book is not for you.

Bullies and those who want to hurt others typically do not excel in the martial arts for the simple reason that skill in the martial arts requires the kind of discipline, strength of character, big-heartedness, and compassion for others that are often lacking in bullies. There are exceptions to this. Some styles that just focus on combat or competition can attract these sorts of bad students, and, if they are sufficiently disciplined, as in any challenging sport, these students might be able to excel.

But this is completely foreign to the spirit of the martial arts. Such students, if they don't change their ways, often end up in prison or in the grave. And this leads me to my first *Tip for Beginners* . . . .

Tip #1:
Don't Pursue the Martial Arts
if you Want to Hurt Others

I remember one time asking one of my instructors if he recommended that I carry a knife for self-defense. I had already had a decade of martial arts training under my belt, and had been given extensive knife fighting and knife self-defense training from this instructor, who had also taught these same skills to elite military forces in the U.S. and across the globe. He himself carried a knife at all times, and usually a handgun on his person, and a shotgun in his car.

In addition to his prowess in unarmed combat (undefeated national full contact champion, three tenth degree black belts, founder of his own system, trainer of elite forces), he was also exceptional in explosives and marksmanship (which he had occasion to use as a contract agent for the U.S. Federal government for special operations at home and abroad that were very dangerous).

His advice to me was NOT to carry a knife! I was surprised. We had spent the last year working almost exclusively on honing my knife fighting and disarming skills, and here he was now telling me NOT to carry a knife for self-defense? When I asked for an explanation, he said that while a knife can be useful under certain rare self-defense circumstances, it's usually just a hazard.

The chances were, he continued, that I would never be in a situation where I would have to physically defend myself— unfortunately, he was wrong there, regardless of my "chances," I did find myself in situations where I had to defend myself. Even if I did have to defend myself, he continued, the chances were that I would not need a knife and probably wouldn't use it even if I had it.

He was correct there, at least so far, as of the writing of this booklet. But he went even further. His concern was twofold. His main concern was that if I carried a knife with me, I might be tempted to escalate a situation, supported by the overconfidence that comes with carrying a lethal weapon, when instead it would be better for me to walk away.

That concern included the worry that regardless of one's skill, the unexpected can always happen, in which case you might get seriously injured or die. Even if I survived the encounter, if I had to use the knife, it would be likely that I would end up in prison. So, I followed his advice, and have never carried a knife around with me on my person, even though I have had to defend myself against knife wielding opponents on a very few occasions.

Why do I share this story? Because, in my experience, my instructor's sage advice has proven true with all of the "bullies" I have known who pursued martial arts. They may not have carried knives or guns on their person—although some of them did—but they carried their martial arts training with them, which can be as deadly.

In all of the instances of "bullies" that stuck with the martial arts and gained lethal skills, they either ended up killed or in prison . . . ALL of them! They picked fights, and sometimes lost their lives in those fights. On other occasions they defended themselves legitimately, but in situations in which they should probably have walked away.

In some of those situations they lost their lives, whereas in others they took lives or severely maimed their opponents, and ended up in prison.

So, if you want to learn martial arts because you want revenge or you want to hurt others, or to be a more "effective" bully, my advice is to seek counselling, to get some serious help, some therapy, but not the martial arts. I don't recommend counselling in a sarcastic way, I mean it sincerely.

Again, in my experience, when someone is mean-spirited, there's usually a reason. I concede that I have seen perhaps three bullies be turned around from the martial arts. In one of those cases, his "conversion" was due to a religious conversion. In the other two instances, it had far more to do with their incredible instructor than the study of martial arts. So, if you want to hurt others, **Don't Pursue Martial Arts!**

Tip #2:
Find a Good Teacher/School:

This second tip is essential. It is so essential, in fact, that I have a forthcoming booklet just devoted to how to find a good teacher and a good school. Moreover, this is not always easy, because you might live in a part of the U.S. or the globe where there simply is no good teacher or school to be found. If all you have is a bad teacher, or bad teachers, or a bad school, then I would recommend postponing your martial arts study until you relocate. Better not to learn martial arts at all than to learn it from a bad teacher of from a bad school.

But how do you know if you have a bad teacher or not? Just watch the first "Karate Kid" movie where Daniel visits the Karate dojo for the first time, and then again later with Mr. Miyagi. That will give you a visceral sense of what a bad school and a bad teacher is like. Of course, you might not be able to figure this out at first. There are some telltale signs, however, that, if not infallible, are at least good indicators that you should just leave:

1) When the instructor tries to strong arm you, bully you, or pressure you like a car salesman to sign up for a long-term contract (a year or more) to their program without any trial lessons or trial period.

2) When the school has absolutely no children's program. This is not always a good indicator. For example, if you instructor only teaches part time, and focuses on an adult program perhaps due to space, liability, time constraints, etc. That's not always bad. If, however, you have a full-time martial arts school, with a full-time instructor, and there are no kids programs, that is usually a bad sign.

3) When the school has no women at all—and this goes for all potential students, men and women alike—run, do not walk, away from that school. In general, women have an interest in self-defense, getting in shape, etc., just as much, and sometimes even more so, than men. This varies somewhat region by region, but is fairly universal, at least in the English-speaking world. If there are no women there at all, there's a good chance that this is not due to the fact that no women have ever looked into that school or instructor, but rather is more likely to the fact that they don't feel comfortable there. I promise you that if women don't feel comfortable there, then neither will you.

4) When the school is immaculately clean—unless it's either very new, or it's not used full time, or it's carpeted or wooden floors, etc. If it has mats—and this is especially the case for martial arts schools that teach Aikido, Brazilian Jiu-Jitsu, any of the traditional Japanese or American JuJutsu styles, Judo, or Mixed Martial Arts. If it's a full-time school, not brand-spanking new (or newly renovated or relocated), then this is a sign that it doesn't get much use. Not the kind of place you want to train.

5) When the school is absolutely filthy. That's probably a sign that the instructors are not very good. Why? Because if they don't care about taking care of the school, they probably don't care much more about taking care of the style, teaching, or students either. This may not always be the case, but it has been in my experience.

6) When the school is overly commercialized. Every martial arts school, especially if it is a full-time school with a full-time instructor, will have some commercial aspects. The school has to stay open, after all, and the instructor has to make a living. That's fine. There's nothing wrong with advertisements, paying for programs, seminars, equipment, videos, etc. This is all standard fare for most full-time martial arts schools. The problem is when it's overly commercialized. If you're expected to buy products with every lesson, and there's no end in sight, then the school is over commercialized.

7) When the instructor refuses to ever say anything positive about other martial arts styles or instructors. That's a definite bad sign. The best instructors I have studied under were supremely confident in their own abilities. They had proven themselves time and again. Moreover, they had lots of options of styles in which to train, and all of them trained in multiple styles over their lives. But they chose the style in which they excelled in because they thought it was the BEST for them. And yet, each of these instructors had many fine things to say about other instructors and other styles. In fact, I can't think of any of my best instructors saying a negative word about any other martial arts instructor—and this even of the instructors who would send students to challenge their students or deface the school's property, which happened on occasion—nor a negative word about any other martial arts style.

8) When the instructor continually brags about their own abilities and experiences when they teach class or are teaching you privately, that's a bad sign. It's a sign that they really don't have that much self-confidence, and that perhaps some of their accolades are made up.

9) When the students are mean-spirited. Here I'm not talking about the occasional student you run across that's just a jerk. I mean the tone or atmosphere of the place—again, see "The Karate Kid." If the students are jerks, the instructor is probably a jerk, or else has no control over her or his students. Either way, not the kind of place you want to be. This is why trial lessons and observing classes in advance can be so important.

There's far more to selecting an instructor and a school, but this is an initial list of **where not to train**. Part of what you're going to want to figure out is what style is best for you. I have a forthcoming booklet devoted to that topic as well. This can be a tricky topic.

Much depends on your goal, and as much depends on your geographical location and finances. If your goal is simply physical fitness, or self-discipline, or self-control, or self-confidence, than practically any martial arts style will do. If you want self-defense, then, most styles would also be sufficient, in terms of long term sufficiency.

What I mean by that is if you spend fifteen or twenty years mastering a style, just about any style, then you will likely be able to defend yourself about as well as any other skilled practitioner. Why? Because, on the one hand, when it comes to deadly weapons like knives, guns, chains, multiple attackers, etc., anything can happen, even to the best of martial artists. I never left the few situations in which I was attacked with a bladed object without getting cut.

Now, I don't claim to be a martial arts master, but four of my teachers who were true masters have also been attacked by knives (and two of them by guns), and all of them were cut when attacked by knives. In fact, the one teacher I mentioned at the beginning of this booklet, who advised me against carrying a knife, had been shot twice, and knifed more times than I can count, and he has the scars to prove it, and this despite having earned three tenth degree black belts, and being an undefeated full contact champion.

In real self-defense, anything can happen. Even the best martial arts masters can be injured, put in the hospital, and killed. That's just real life. If you show up to a school and that instructor tells you they can make you an invincible weapon that either their style or their instruction and training will ensure your survival in a real self-defense situation, or enable you to defend yourself in any situation unscathed, run!!! You may learn some useful skills, but you will be gaining a dangerous (indeed LETHAL) misplaced confidence that will likely get you hurt and may get you killed.

That being said, regardless of the style in which you train, you will be getting in better physical shape—stronger, greater endurance, more power, more flexibility, greater awareness of threats and of your surroundings, speed, agility, etc. These will all better enable you to defend yourself, or know when and how to flee and avoid a situation.

Finally, if you've spent fifteen or twenty years in a style, you'll have a good grasp of that style, and you'll have a stockpile of techniques that work best for you—that you've practiced the most, that come to you naturally, that fit your body size, etc., and that you're fairly effective at using.

So much of self-defense in the real world amounts to avoidance, knowing how to get away or creating the ability to get away, or taking the attacker by surprise—they don't expect any resistance or they wouldn't have attacked you in the first place. In another forthcoming booklet we'll cover the essentials of self-defense. The point is, that if that's your goal, and if you're not in a rush, virtually any style will do. If you're in a rush, then you'll have to narrow down styles a bit, and we'll cover this more in my forthcoming booklet on how to choose which martial arts style is best for you.

The short answer as to martial arts style you should choose is going to be easier to determine based on the your answers to the following questions:

1) What martial arts styles are available in the nearby areas that you're willing and able to travel to? You'll have to ask yourself how far you are willing and able to go to get instruction? That's the first way to narrow down the martial art that you should train in. If you live in a densely populated area, perhaps a city, or are willing to commute rather far, say an hour or two each way to train, then you'll have a lot more options open to you.

2) What times/days of the week are you willing and able to take classes/lessons, and which styles are available with those times/days as options? Some of you might want to try to train every day. You should certainly try to practice every day, if you can.

Training every day, learning and being corrected by an instructor, is not necessary, although it can be beneficial. Sometimes, depending on the style, just a few days a week is sufficient. Or, especially for more advanced students in styles like Kung Fu or Ninjutsu, once a week or once a month is sufficient, so long as you are practicing most days. It all depends on the style, your goals, and your availability.

3) What schools/instructors are in your price range. Sometimes prices for classes or private instruction are available on the school's website. Other times you might ask one of the students if you know anyone who trains at the school in question. You should always ask the school, and can usually call them.

Sometimes schools will be hesitant to list the price for a variety of reasons. Sometimes they just don't want to scare away potential students because prices might be high and they think that some students, after a trial period, will be hooked and willing and able to pay whereas, had they initially heard the price without having tried it out, they would have been scared away.

Other times, they don't want to mention the price because they might have various payment options open but need to find out how much the potential student is willing and able to pay—the schools and instructors don't want to get cheated by potential students either. Other times, there's something fishy going on. Just be aware that if a school is hesitant to discuss prices before trial lessons, this is not necessarily a bad sign. At the same time, some schools/instructors simply might be out of your price range.

4) Once you've limited the possibilities by distance and time slots, and perhaps finances, it's time to eliminate schools by the nine criteria I listed above on what to avoid in a school/instructor. Sometimes you'll be able to eliminate schools on these criteria before even getting to the prices.

For others, you'll have so many options after location and times to train, and perhaps even prices, and you can't just try out all of the schools left on the list . . . . I mean, you might still have a Mixed Martial Arts school, Brazilian Jiu-Jitsu, Israeli Krav Maga, Tae Kwon Do, Tang Soo Do, Hapkido, Aikido, Ninjutsu, Shotokan Karate, Goju-ryu Karate, Tiger Claw Kung Fu, Wing Chun, Jeet Kune Do, Norther Shaolin Kung Fu, Tai Chi, Fitness Kickboxing, Judo, Daito-ryu Jujutsu, Kenpo Karate, some new American style, etc., all within those remaining criteria. So which should you choose?

In my forthcoming booklet, we'll go through the major styles available in the U.S. and must of Europe as well, to help you make that decision. For now, it depends a lot on your goals. Here's a sample of what I mean:

If you just want to get into shape, learn some techniques that you can use to defend yourself on the street, gain self-confidence and self-discipline, then any of these styles could do. You might just want to start reading about the styles in your area online and see if any catch your interest, and/or start showing up to the schools and see which strikes your fancy.

If you want to go into competition fighting, Mixed Martial Arts seems to be the thing, but it depends on what kind of competition you want. If you want old school Karate style competitions, like those that made action star Chuck Norris initially famous, than any Karate style, or Korean style like Tae Kwon Do, would do just fine. There are a number of Kung Fu fighting competitions available too, from San Shou to Kuoshu and other competitions—and you could still fight in an MMA context (although I'd recommend learning Chinese grappling like Shuai Jiao if that's the case).

If you're a police officer and want to learn restraining techniques that won't get you in trouble, I'd probably recommend Aikido, even though MMA and Brazilian Jiu-Jitsu are very popular among police, and Aikido takes many years to master. The reason, in my opinion, is that Aikido contains the locks and holds of traditional Jujutsu, but its whole focus is using the opponent's energy against them, to do as little damage as possible.

A master of Brazilian Jiu-Jitsu can do this too, but Brazilian Jiu-Jitsu was forged in one-on-one challenge matches in the streets and beaches of Brazil. One of its signature finishing moves has your back on the ground, your opponent's back against your chest, as you choke them out.

Very effective in MMA style matches, but it doesn't protect you very well against other potential opponents (who are potentially armed) in the surrounding areas, which Police officers always have to worry about, and, moreover, so many of those martial techniques are illegal for police to use, at least in the U.S. Aikido, on the other hand, turns deadly Jujutsu chokes, into throws (which could be equally deadly on concrete and for the opponent who doesn't know how to fall safely), but the Aikido throws can be turned, quite easily, into even less dangerous restraints.

If you're training for potential hand-to-hand combat scenarios in a military setting, where you might be willing to blind, otherwise maim, or kill an opponent when your gun, or knife has failed, than perhaps Krav Maga, or a traditional Japanese or American style of Jujutsu or synthetic Karate might be a good complement (or even superior to) what you receive in your regular military training. Of course, probably any style will be a nice complement to your military training, and might even provide you with more options in combat. I'm just giving you a few examples.

If you want a lot of kicking techniques, Aikido is not for you. Wing Chun is probably not for you. Nor Brazilian Jiu-Jitsu. If you really want to do lots of diverse kicking techniques, try a traditional Korean style like Tae Kwon Do, or Tang Soo Do, or a northern style of Kung Fu, or Muay Thai, or even a traditional Okinawan or Japanese Karate style.

If you want a lot of grappling, try Judo, or wrestling, or Mixed Martial Arts, or Brazilian Jiu-Jitsu. If you want to learn a lot of weaponry try any traditional Kung Fu style (although some, like Wing Chun, only use a few weapons), or Ninjutsu, or Okinawan or Japanese Karate styles. It all depends on what your goals are. You have to determine that and then find the best school/instructor you can.

In some instances, I would go against common wisdom and suggest learning a style, even if it's a bit more expensive (but still within your price range) that you might not have studied otherwise, precisely because of the instructor.

So, for example, even though I have studied both southern and northern styles of Chinese Kung Fu, I personally prefer the northern styles. Part of this is a matter of taste. For me, personally, I enjoy practicing northern Kung Fu forms more than I do southern style forms. Northern styles tend to have more kicking and flowery techniques. I also like norther pole forms (like long staff and spear) better than their southern counterparts. This is just a matter of personal taste. I'm in no way trying to say anything negative about southern Kung Fu styles.

That being said, if I lived near a Grandmaster of a small southern style, and he personally taught at some small school—all things being equal, I would study under him rather than under some newly-minted black sash who studied under a Sifu who studied under a Sifu who studied under a Sifu who studied under the current Grandmaster of that style, even if it was a northern style I prefer, like one of the Praying Mantis styles I've studied. So these are all things to keep in mind.

You might not want to study Ninjutsu, but if you discovered you lived near a great Ninjutsu master who was willing to teach you, and you had no problem studying Ninjutsu, then that might be what you'd want to study.

Tip #3:
Train Hard, but Not Too Hard:

This can be tricky. You want to train hard, to push yourself, but you don't want to injure yourself. Chances are, you're going to get bruises, perhaps scrapes, and minor injuries like these, regardless of what style you study, even the internal Chinese styles like Tai Chi and Hsingi-I can involve bruises, if you practice Tai Chi pushing hands, or do any sort of technique work beyond solo forms. And of course if you're using weapons (and this certainly goes for Tai Chi, Hsing-I, and Pa Kua), your muscles will get sore.

If you take up Brazilian Jiu-Jitsu, MMA, etc., then sometimes more serious injuries occur as well, just as they do in wrestling and boxing. In general, however, you want to try to avoid injuries. This requires that you take the time to warm up and stretch your muscles.

Most traditional styles come with their own warm up routine, and what I've found is that each style's warm up routine relates to the actual techniques and type of practice in the style. So, when I studied Kung Fu, the warm up routines, I've since discovered, are perfect to prepare one for practicing Kung Fu forms and weapons routines. That makes sense since that is the bulk of what our practice consisted of.

When I studied Tai Chi or Hsing-I, the warm up routines helped limber up lightly, and also facilitated the spread of Chi throughout the body. Again, that makes sense for the type of training. When I studied Aikido, classes were primarily composed of practicing techniques—two to four per class—most of which involved throwing, and being thrown, on the mat. So, our warm ups focused on loosening up, especially stretching the back (not so much the hamstrings, since we weren't going to be doing any kicking), the ankles, the knees, and of course, practice falling and rolling on our own.

Again, these warm ups prepared us for the practice sessions. So, take your time and warm up properly. Moreover, get to know your physical ability, if you have injuries, an illness, old age, if you're new to the practice of martial arts, etc. All of these factors can help you in determining how far to go in practice.

If you can't do certain things, let your instructor know, as well as the partners you'll be training with. If it's a good school, no one will have a problem with this. If they have a problem with it, then you need to find a new school. It can be humbling to let people know they have to go a little easier on you, or not throw you to the ground because of a back or knee injury, or simply because of your age. But you need to take these precautions so that you don't get injured.

Usually, the younger you are, the more you can probably push yourself and get away with it. If you're new to martial arts, or just getting back into it after a long hiatus, be careful for the first few weeks. You're bound to get very sore and in places you're not used to being sore, for several weeks, perhaps a month or two, or more. Just keep with it. It will be important to learn to distinguish muscle soreness, and slight bruising, from strained, sprained, and pulled muscles, tendons, and ligaments.

Tip #4:
Eat Well:

     This may sound like a strange tip, but in my experience, what you eat is one of the most important factors in how well you train and even in how you feel. You want to eat sufficient calories to perform the exercise well, even if you're trying to lose weight. If you're trying to lose weight, you need to burn more calories than you consume, but you still need sufficient calories to burn, or else you will be prone to injury. Eating a well-balanced diet, with plenty of vitamins and minerals, is essential. Sure you'll need some carbs and protein, but at least in the U.S., we tend to get more than we need of carbs and protein. You may also want to invest in some dietary supplements to make sure you're getting enough vitamins and minerals. You'll probably need more than you naturally get in food, unless you already eat exceptionally healthily.

Tip #5:
Keep Well-Hydrated:

This should be a no-brainer, but I can't tell you how many times I've seen people pass out in training in part from lack of hydration and loss of salt. Water is essential, and sometimes sports drinks that replace electrolytes in addition, but always water first and foremost.

Tip #6:
Practice Outside of Class:

To gain skill in your martial arts training, you must practice outside of class. If you're just trying to get in shape, and you're showing up to three or four classes a week, you might not need much practice outside of class, but you should at least put in a little exercise outside of class, even if that only amounts to walking and stretching.

If you really want to gain skill in your style, however, you must practice outside of class. I would go so far as to say that you must practice more than you train . . . far more! What do I mean by this? Well, when you train you are being taught and/or corrected. When you practice, you hone your skills, becoming progressively more proficient.

When I trained with my Karate instructor once a week in private lessons, he would teach me one technique, and one technique only, that week. We would go over the technique for about an hour. Then I would spend at least an hour a day every day for that next week, practicing the technique I learned.

It is in the practice and the repetitions that we really burn those techniques into our muscle memory. That is where real skill develops. Of course we need to continue to be corrected on the techniques, to get all the fine points and precisions right. This is even more the case with Kata routines, or Kung Fu forms and weapons training. Practicing on our own and with a partner is where we really get good.

Tip #7:
Video-tape Yourself Training:

For some reason, most martial artists I know don't videotape themselves, despite the fact that they have Ipads, Smart Phones, computers, etc., with all of this technology available to them. When I studied Aikido, we not only practiced the techniques, the throws, but also receiving the techniques, the falling. This helped because it taught us how to do the techniques not only by doing them, but by having them done to us.

When I studied Goshin-Jitsu, we had a mirror in which we watched ourselves performing the techniques. This was helpful, so we could see if we were performing the technique like the instructor. When I studied Karate, at the end of each class, I wrote down in a notebook all the details of the technique covered so that I could go back to my notebook later and make sure I was doing the technique correctly.

In this new age of technology, however, I film myself. No, I don't post these films. No, I don't sell them. They're just for me. I've enough experience in the styles in which I still practice, especially my American Karate style, that I film my practice every day. Then, at the end of the week, I spend time looking over the films.

This takes time, but I start to notice, "woops, I dropped my hand there . . . . Oh, no, that wasn't a 45 degree angle . . . . Oh, gosh, I should have been aiming for where their throat was, but instead, that would have been my opponent's chest." Then I can take a few notes, and really work on improving the techniques that may have atrophied over the years.

You might not be as advanced yet, but what you can see is where what you're doing is not what you're instructor was doing. When you're practicing a technique, like as a beginner in Aikido for instance, you might need to keep your arms more extended than they are.

You might think they're extended, and yet, in the video you can see they're too collapsed. After a decade or more of Aikido practice, you might be very powerful with short techniques, but especially in the beginning of Aikido, you want to make everything as extended as possible, unless your Sensei tells you otherwise.

Tip #8:
Just Practice One Martial Art
at a Time
as a Beginner:

I've studied numerous martial arts . . . too many in fact. Part of the reason for all of the styles I've studied is that I moved around a lot over these past thirty years. It's better to gain proficiency, mastery, of one style than to have some knowledge of many. I have some knowledge of many.

I concede I have some proficiency in some of them, but no mastery. At least, not mastery in my book, and I've worked with many masters. My instructors have been 4th, 5th, and 7th degree black belts in Aikido, a 10th degree black belt in Karate and two different styles of Jujutsu, 5th, 6th, 7th, and 8th degree black sashes in Kung Fu, etc.

My recommendation would be stick with one style. The exceptions would be complementary styles. So, if you practice a northern style of Kung Fu, it could be very beneficial to study Tai Chi as well, and perhaps Shuai Jiao if you're physically able, and of course Chin-Na.

If you study Aikido, it could be a very good idea to study some form of Japanese swordsmanship, since so much of Aikido originated with the sword, putting the sword into the empty hand throws. So you might want to take up Kendo, or a specific Kenjutsu style besides the Aiki Ken that comes built in with most Aikido practice (at least at the advanced level), or Iaido.

But, it's probably not very helpful to practice Tae Kwon Do and Tang Soo Do at the same time, unless you've already mastered one. If you're a black belt in one style, then perhaps you can add another style.

Tip #9:
Learn to Take Correction Well:

Don't feel bad when you are corrected by your instructor, or be a classmate who either outranks you or who has been training longer than you. In fact, even if a junior classmate corrects you, so long as you're not certain they're the one making a beginner's mistake, such corrections can greatly help you.

Be respectful and take the corrections to heart. Your attitude should be, "Corrections? The more the merrier." Don't think that corrections mean that you're a poor martial artist or that there's no hope for you. Think instead that each correction is only making you an even better martial artist.

Tip #10:
Teach,
When You can:

    Teach some of what you learn, prudentially, to friends or family that you trust. The reasons are many: it can give you someone else to practice with outside of official classes; teaching helps you learn the material better; and you can help others by teaching them the martial arts.

    When should you begin doing this? Well, when in doubt, as your instructor? I think a good rule of thumb is that after you've made it to a higher rank, you might be able to teach some of the basics of the previous rank to someone else . . . at least you should be able to.

    You won't have the finesse or precision of a black belt/black sash. So, don't charge money. Moreover, don't teach in such a way that you're asserting yourself as master. Also be careful who you teach.

    You don't want to teach someone who will be a bully. Look at it as a practice opportunity for you. Makes sure the environment is safe. Go slow.

    Work on precision and skill, not speed, not strength, not effectiveness of technique.

Just work on the basics, until you gain some level of proficiency. Be very careful and always err on the side of caution.

Tip #11:
Read as Much as You Can on the Style You're Studying:

The more you know about your style, the more interest you'll maintain, the more you'll assist your perseverance with training and practice, and the more you'll understand what you are practicing. Thus, the more you read, the better you'll get, all things being equal—nutrition, rest, practice, etc.

Tip #12:
Set Goals
***for Yourself*:**

You should frequently be making goals and resolutions for yourself, not only to keep you motivated, but to have concrete goals in mind to help you progress along the way. They can be as simple as preparing for an upcoming ranking exam to move to the next level, or a certain level of repetitions of a technique (one hundred sword cuts each day), or learning a particular technique or form, etc. Set goals frequently, and take the necessary steps to meeting those goals.

Tip #13:
Vary Your Practice
to Avoid Overtraining
and
to Keep Interested:

You probably don't want to cross train with aerobics everyday, nor with weights, although both can be beneficial. Whatever your style, you should be careful not to over train.

If you're an advanced Kung Fu practitioner, maybe you'll work on empty hand forms three or four days a week, two or three each time. Maybe you'll practice weapons three times a week. Perhaps if you're learning a new weapon, or a new form, you'll do least a few good repetitions (not for exercise but for precision—to get it right not to break a sweat) 7 days a week.

But a few days a week, two, three, or four, you'll run through the form, as well as some others that you don't want to forget, a hundred times or more.

Obviously you'll have to work up to this. Perhaps Monday will be the day you work with the short staff, long staff, and spear. Perhaps Wednesday will be the day for straight sword, broadsword, and double broadsword. Perhaps Friday will be your day for Kwan Dao, Da Dao.

If you're working on learning the Three Section Staff, perhaps you'll work on that a little each day, or before you're flexible weapons like rope dart and nine section steel whip.

Tip #14:
Don't Take Yourself Too Seriously—
Be Comfortable with Failure:

The final tip, learn to fail well. Don't take yourself too seriously. Even on a test, it's ok to fail. The failures don't have the final say. Rather, it's your perseverance that will have the final say.

The greatest masters aren't the ones who never made mistakes or failed. As is has become cliché, they're the ones who failed and made more mistakes than the rest of us have even tried.

So fail and fail away. Learn from your failures. Try again. Don't give up. Of course you'll fail and make more mistakes than you'll ever be able to keep track of.

Think of me with my videos of myself, even after nearly thirty years of training and practice: "woops . . . I could have done that better." That's the idea. Beginning the martial arts is embarking on a life of life-long improvement in an art that's martial.

There's a lethal beauty in each martial art that's uniquely its own. Find one to train in, and you'll become a better person, with more confidence and skill. Fall in love with one, and you'll have a life-long activity to keep you healthy and safe for the rest of your life.

Please check out my martial arts blog, Pat Smith Martial Arts, at
patsmithmartialarts.wordpress.com,
for more information on the martial arts and my new writing projects.

About the Author:

Pat Smith has nearly thirty years' experience in the martial arts. He studied a variety of martial arts styles including Chinese, Japanese, Korean, and American styles.

Pat's broadest experience is in the Chinese styles. He studied a variety of the internal styles of Chinese martial arts that aid health and well-being as well prove to be quite devastating in combat: Chi Kung, Hsing-I Chuan, Pa Kua Chang, and Tai Chi Chuan. He also studied a number of different Kung Fu styles: Monkey style, various Northern Praying Mantis styles, Northern Shaolin, Sun Pin, and Wing Chun. His Chinese training included weapons training. In addition, he studied the Chinese grappling arts of Chin-Na and Shuai Jiao.

His experience in the Korean arts includes Tang Soo Do and Tae Kwon Do. The majority of his training in Japanese styles has been in Aikido and Aikijujutsu. His primary American training is in a rare synthetic Karate style from the Midwest which resembles a combination of Mixed Martial Arts and Israeli Krav Maga, a style tailor made for vicious street self-defense as well as for military and security hand-to-hand combat.

Pat has taught Aikijujutsu, Chin-Na, Hsing-I, Kung Fu, the exclusive American synthetic style, and other arts, to select private students. Pat also hosts a martial arts blog, Pat Smith Martial Arts, patsmithmartialarts.wordpress.com. And check out my Facebook page. You can also follow me on Twitter @PatSmithMartial.

If you enjoyed this resources, make sure to check out my other electronic resources from Amazon.com:

Secrets of Kung Fu Mastery: The Fundamentals

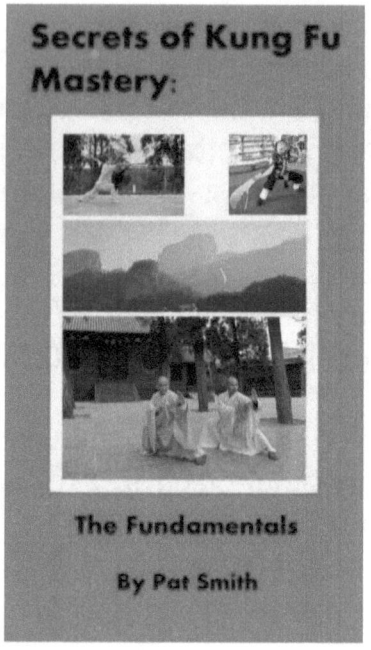

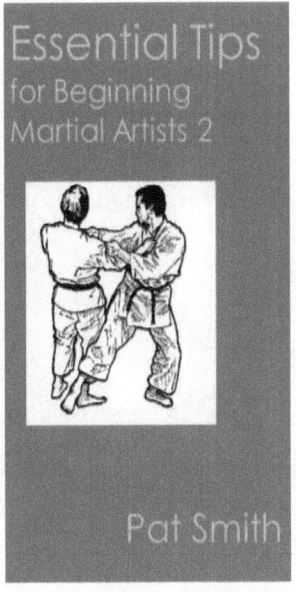

Palm Stick Self-Defense Guide: What to Look for in this Devastating & Practical Defense Tool

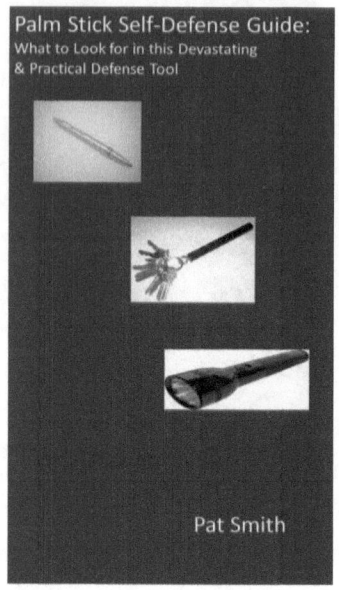

And

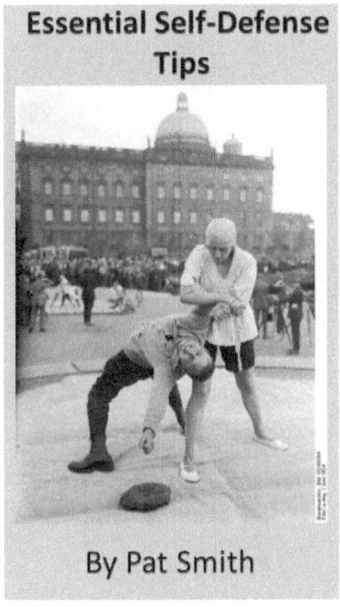